Driving Tips for Senior Drivers

Copyright 2014, Greg Pospiel

This book is dedicated to my wife Debbie, my son Gregory and to my wonderful parents John and Jennie.

Introduction

According to the NHTSA nearly 50,000 accidents between 2007 and 2010 were due to a drivers prior medical condition including: seizures, blackouts, diabetes, heart attack, and stroke! According to the National Institute on Aging: older drivers face a number of challenges. As we age, we begin to gradually develop a multitude of problems that not only affect our overall health but can slow down our reflexes, motor skills, impair our judgment and reaction time and dull our senses. *Our vision starts to go; especially our night vision, glare becomes an issue, our hearing becomes less than perfect, our muscles begin to ache causing our reflexes to slow, we can slowly develop memory loss, numerous medical conditions from obesity to heart disease, type 2 diabetes etc.; we may be taking numerous medications each of which can also lead to side effects such as drowsiness, blurred vision and a host of other issues that can dull our senses and our reaction time to even the most routine driving situations.* We all know someone whether it's grandma, grandpa or an aging parent or sibling who doesn't drive quite the same as they used to. Not only do we see it in their driving but they may be forced to use walking aids, hearing aids, bifocal glasses, they keep the TV volume cranked up high and can't seem to hear anyone on the telephone. Sound familiar?

This material will not only open our minds to the changes taking place in our bodies but also help significantly increase our awareness and should assist in improving our driving skills. Even the most experienced driver develops not only some health issues but also some bad habits like driving too fast, rolling through stop signs, following too close, not checking mirrors and blind spots and blocking traffic in order to make a turn. We tend to forget the rules of the road and make them up as we go along which can significantly increase our chances of having a motor vehicle accident.

Every driver needs to have skill and confidence, command and control of his or her vehicle and awareness of his or her surroundings including road hazards, traffic, and pedestrians.

Remember that in this modern age of technology; cell phones and other distractions have caused countless fatalities. Turn your cell phone off but have it on hand for emergencies and don't focus on watching your GPS, let your passenger keep an eye on it for you.

Table of Contents

Introduction

Some Bad Habits of Older Drivers

General driving tips

Special driving situations

Safety First!

Maneuvers

Things to Remember

What To Do if You're Involved In an Accident

Some Bad Habits of Older Drivers

- Not being aware of our medications and their side effects
- Not wearing your seatbelt
- Making dangerous or last minute maneuvers
- A lack of awareness of your surroundings
- Forgetting to signal for turns, when pulling over, when leaving the side of the road, when parallel parking or in and out of a three point turn
- Forgetting to check mirrors and blind spots for traffic and pedestrians when changing lanes or backing
- Not yielding to or blocking traffic when turning
- Not yielding to school buses or emergency vehicles
- Difficulty performing maneuvers such as being unable to parallel park successfully
- Traffic light violations
- Speed violations

- Poor Judgment when it comes to safe distance between cars, in parking spaces etc.
- Blocking cross walks and intersections

General Practice Tips If You Haven't Driven for A While

- Review the rules of the road and traffic signs
- Know how to operate the brakes, gas, and steering wheel as well as the instrument panel controls such as signals, horn, hazards, wipers and defrosters
- Drive in a variety of settings and conditions progressing from side roads to rural winding roads, one-lane roads, to multi lane and secondary roads and once you're up to it, interstate highways
- Start by focusing on the basics; hand over hand turning, steering control, brake and gas control, making smooth right and left turns, safe stops, right of way at intersections, etc. You may want to start by going around the block making right turns and then reverse direction

making left turns until you are comfortable with the process. Unless you are stopped at a stop sign or traffic light, you'll usually want to add just enough brake to control the turn, perform the hand over hand technique, hold the wheel as the car turns, straighten out and smoothly apply the gas
- Practice driving on city streets, multi lane roads, lane changes, turns using left and right turn lanes at controlled intersections

Once you become comfortable with the basics, move on to practicing maneuvers such as securing the vehicle, backing in a straight line, three point turns, hill starts, parallel, perpendicular and angle parking.

General Driving Tips- A quick look at some things you probably already know!

Hand Position-

The generally accepted position is the 10 and 2 position just like on the hands of a clock. You should always keep two hands on the wheel except when doing hand over hand turns, as you will have to alternate the hand you are using to turn the wheel.

Hand Over Hand Turning –

This gives some drivers difficulty in the beginning. Think of it as alternating hands.

If turning left, start with your hands in the 10 and 2 positions; bring your right hand around to the left hand position, then move the left hand up to the right hand position, bring it over to the left hand position and continue alternating hands as needed. Don't try to keep both hands on the wheel when doing this and don't make too many turns, usually two or three turns is enough. Once the car is in the turn, hold the wheel there until the car makes a complete 90 degree turn then slowly and smoothly bring the wheel back to the center position and bring your hands back to the driving position; accelerate smoothly as you come out of the turn and the car straightens out. Try not to use too much gas going into a turn. Work on this until it becomes one smooth motion.

Blind Spots-

Your blind spot is almost right next to you, just slightly to the backside of your car. Check your rear view mirror then your side mirror and blind spot when changing lanes, leaving the side of the roadway or backing up. You can identify your blind spot while parked on the side of the road by looking at passing cars in your side mirror and note when they disappear from view, then note how long it takes for the car to come into your peripheral (side) vision; you might be surprised to find that it's only a fraction of a second. Constantly scan your mirrors while driving as the traffic is constantly changing.

Speed Control-

While you want to be careful of not going over the speed limit, going too slow can be just as bad and can also cause confusion and accidents. Stay with the speed limit and traffic flow unless conditions or weather call for slower speeds. Also be careful not to go too slow in your turns, use your brake as needed to control the car through the turn but avoid stopping midway as this can cause an accident.

Controlled Intersections -

If the light turns yellow at an intersection, you should stop if it is safe to do so. Be aware of your speed and distance from the intersection; the closer you are to the intersection or the higher your speed, the more difficult it will be to stop safely. This will become easier with practice and experience.

When the light turns green be aware of traffic that may still be going through the intersection. If there are vehicles ahead of you, give them a second to go to make sure they proceed through the intersection and don't decide to slam on their brakes due to traffic or pedestrians. This causes countless accidents because everyone is in such a rush to go when the light turns green.

Stop Signs-

Make full stops at stop signs; check traffic in both directions before proceeding.

Green Arrow-

A green arrow on a left turn means you have a protected turn; if there is no arrow and the light turns green, you must wait for oncoming traffic to clear before proceeding with your left turn.

No Turn On Red -

Be aware of no turn on red signs and make a complete stop before turning right on red where it is allowed.

Flashing lights -

Flashing yellow means watch for traffic and proceed with caution.

Flashing red lights mean stop - the same as a stop sign.

Remember if you have a flashing red, the cross traffic probably has a flashing yellow or caution in which case they are not obligated to stop.

Uncontrolled Intersections -

At an uncontrolled intersection - one without a traffic control device yield to any cars already in the intersection. If two cars arrive at the same time, the driver to the left must yield to the driver to the right. If it's your turn to go don't hesitate too long; this causes confusion and accidents.

T Intersections -

At a T intersection, the through traffic has right of way as you are turning into traffic.

Roundabouts and Rotaries -

Always yield to traffic that is already in the rotary as well as bicycles and pedestrians. Signal right to exit.

Right Turns –

Signal to alert other drivers. When there is no stop sign present, avoid stopping in your turn, but slow down by braking smoothly - only enough brake as is needed to control the turn, stay in the closest lane, come out a few feet to clear the curb and be aware of parked cars that you may have to go around. As you complete your turn straighten the wheel and gradually accelerate. If traveling uphill you may need less brake and slightly give more gas as you complete the turn. Don't forget to check for no turn on red signs and check for traffic and pedestrians.

Left Turns -

Signal first, check for traffic and move into the left lane or left turn lane if on a multi lane road. (If you have trouble making left turns - picture a large truck sitting perpendicular to you in the intersection in the lane to your left and steer around it so that you end up on the right side of the yellow line.) Remember to turn into the closest lane or (right turn/right lane and left turn/left lane) if turning onto a multi lane road. If there are two left turn lanes stay in the lane you are in when you complete the turn.

Avoid pulling out into traffic and blocking oncoming cars in order to make your turn, instead wait at the stop line for an opening. If you have a green light; yield to oncoming traffic, identify an opening, and begin to make your turn if the light is still green. If there are two lanes of traffic one oncoming and one turning left, make sure the oncoming lane is clear before turning. If the oncoming car is turning left and you are turning left it's ok to go just use caution and keep an eye on traffic that may be behind the car that is turning left in case it tries to go around him.

Passing -

The far left lane should be used as a passing lane. Passing on the right is ok if the vehicle ahead is making a left turn assuming there is room for two vehicles in that direction. Passing on the right is also allowed when the other vehicle is on a one-way road and is in the left lane or the lane has construction or perhaps some other type of obstruction.

Avoid passing cars on the left on two lane roads even when you have a broken line as it can quickly become a game of cat and mouse if another vehicle suddenly approaches from the other direction or pulls out of a driveway and you have no room to get back into your lane. A head on collision is not worth the three or four minutes you might have saved by passing the other car. Never attempt to speed up or block a car that is trying to pass as this can lead to a fatal head on collision if there is oncoming traffic.

Brake and Gas Control -

The best advice here is, go easy on the gas and easy on the brake. As you drive and conditions change you will find you need to adjust your speed frequently. Sometimes you will need to brake suddenly, most of the time you will want to slow down gradually and come to a smooth stop. As you go around a curved road you may need to apply some brake to control the car through the turn, then release the brake as you feel you have the car in control, add gas smoothly as you come out of the turn and add more gas if the road starts to go uphill or maybe a little more brake if the road starts to go downhill. Remember not to keep stopping but just use the brake as much as is needed to maintain control. Also, how many times have you heard on the news that an elderly driver stepped on the gas by mistake or drove forward through the window of a café instead of reversing out of the space? An easy fix here is to just look down at the shifter before moving, and tap the gas lightly once before committing to backing out. Once you see the car is going the way you want it to, you're on your way. And always check carefully for traffic and other cars that may be backing out behind you.

Emergency Vehicles –

Look, listen, determine which direction the emergency vehicle is coming from; signal, pull over to the side and stop.

School busses –

Stop when lights are flashing no matter which side the bus is on. (Not needed if there is a Jersey type barrier and the bus is on the opposite side on a divided highway.) Do not proceed until the bus turns off its flashing lights or the bus driver tells you to go.

Special Driving Situations

City driving –

City driving is stop and go; you must be on your game at all times. Expect cars ahead of you to make sudden stops, expect cars to pull out from parking lots, and pedestrians to walk or run across the street. Also watch for taxis, city busses, bicycles, skateboarders, wheelchairs, parked cars, open doors, etc. Leave extra space especially at intersections. When the light turns green, let the car ahead of you proceed for a second or two before accelerating to make sure that the vehicle does not suddenly stop for traffic or pedestrians. Once you're certain the vehicle in front of you is not braking, you can accelerate safely.

Highway Merging –

Check for other cars that may also be entering the on ramp from you right or left, make certain any cars ahead of you on the ramp have left before you accelerate to speed, signal left, get your vehicle up to speed in the acceleration lane, identify an opening in the first lane, yield to highway traffic as needed, check mirror and blind spot before accelerating, accelerate smoothly to the speed of traffic. As you approach an off ramp, start to slow down in the deceleration lane by taking your foot off the gas first, this will slow the car down a bit without causing other cars to have to slam on their brakes, then apply your brake lightly or as needed. Most off ramps are marked between 25 and 35 mph but when exiting, adjust your speed according to traffic, weather and road conditions.

Remember large trucks have blind spots on all sides so it's not a good idea to stay too close. Be aware of cars that may cut in front of you often using no signal especially as you approach an exit ramp as they may be in a rush to get over and make that exit.

Severe weather –

Use headlights, wipers, defrosters as needed, adjust speed to weather, road and traffic conditions, use the brake and gas lightly and slow down early, leave extra space between you and the cars ahead of you. Use light pressure on the gas, brakes and steering wheel to avoid sliding.

In severe weather conditions such as hurricane, tornado, nor'easters, heavy snow and white out conditions, *avoid driving if possible* otherwise, let someone know where you are going and when you expect to get there. Keep an emergency kit with you (blankets, sweaters, hat, gloves, boots, water, protein bars, medications, flashlight, and a flag to mark your car in case you get stranded in snow.) A whistle should also be in your emergency kit. You can use the whistle if you get stranded in your vehicle. Stay in your car and run it every ten minutes or so for heat and to charge your cell phone. While this may sound extreme, driving in bad weather can become a matter of life and death.

When I worked in the insurance industry, I once took a claim from a woman who was on her way home from college when a tornado hit the Springfield, MA area. She saw the tornado coming, parked on the side of the road and hid under her dashboard as it passed over her. A telephone pole was struck by lightning and the pole crashed down on her car, her car burst into flames and she ran out. She said as she ran through the ankle deep water she felt electricity surging through her body. This is real life, emergencies do happen. Be aware of severe weather alerts and if possible, stay off the roads during severe weather. Avoid driving down flooded roads or through flooded areas as the water can rise quickly leaving you trapped in side your vehicle!

Winter Driving-

In the winter be careful of black ice. Black ice is hard to see, it can be a thin film of frozen water that can cause you to lose traction and slide off the road or into oncoming traffic. Use caution; slow down, brake lightly, turn gently; avoid sudden or hard movements.

Winter driving requires preparation as well as care and attention. Pay attention to weather reports and try to avoid travel during the height of a storm. If you must go out, clean the snow off of your roof and every part of your car including the lights. Leave extra space for slowing down; watch for snow removal vehicles, look ahead for hazards such as accidents, black ice, etc. Use your signals and brake early to alert vehicles that may be behind you.

Focus on driving rather than the cell phone, text messaging, the radio and passengers who may be trying to get your attention.

Safety First!

Safety – Avoid driving at night if your vision is starting to become a problem. Plan your route so you are taking roads you're familiar and keep a cell phone nearby in case of an emergency. OnStar is also a great tool to have! Know your medications and all the side effects. Ask your doctor or pharmacist if any of your medications should be avoided prior to driving. Keep up with routine medical exams, eye exams, and closely monitor your diabetes and blood sugar levels to assure you are in top shape for a long trip. Avoid driving if you are feeling sleepy, drowsy, light headed, fatigued or have any other signs that you are not up to the task. Don't be too proud to ask a relative or friend to drive you to the store or a doctor's appointment if you are not up to it.

Always scan the road far ahead for hazards such as accidents, slowing traffic, brake lights and turn signals, busy intersections, driveways, cars that may be pulling out of parking lots, construction zones, emergency vehicles, pedestrians etc. Don't get fixated on the car in front of you. With over six million accidents per year and some two million rear end accidents per year, distance is your best friend. Distance is as important as speed, adjust both for weather and traffic conditions; be sure to leave enough space between cars so that you can safely stop in any emergency. Follow the two and four second rules but keep in mind that two or four seconds is not a lot of time to react so you should constantly be asking yourself if you have enough room to stop or take evasive action in an emergency in the current traffic and weather conditions. Just recently while driving with a student driver, an SUV fell off of a tow truck right in front of us; fortunately we had plenty of distance to slow down and stop but it happened quite fast and if we were too close, the story would have ended much differently.

When an accident happens, cars and car parts such as doors and hoods can go flying out of control, cars can roll over, come flying across center lines; a utility or light pole can come crashing down etc. You will need both time and distance to safely move out of the way, into the breakdown lane, into a grassy area or slow down and stop safely on the shoulder. On highways, remember that accidents happen extremely fast (much like they do in a NASCAR race,) leave as much distance as possible between cars at highway speeds; both cars and trucks can go spinning out of control and bouncing off of guardrails and into other cars ahead of you in just a few short seconds.

You should constantly be asking yourself if you have enough room to stop or move out of the way quickly if the cars ahead of you brake suddenly or go spinning out of control ahead of you. You will need extra space to slow down, move into the break down lane or a grassy area or slow down and stop to avoid hitting any number of careening cars, car parts and trucks.

Always keep escape routes in mind such as the shoulder, grassy areas, exit ramps etc. Avoid driving too close to large trucks; they have blind spots and can also kick up stones that can damage your windshield, even pickup trucks or any large trucks that carry tools or pull trailers such as landscaping trailers can lose tools, stones, ladders and even trailers have been known to come separated from trucks.

Wearing the wrong shoes such as sandals, flip-flops or bulky winter boots can cause an accident. Recently on the news, a driver was wearing sandals and his sandal got caught on the pedal causing his car to go through his garage and land in his in ground swimming pool!

Horn-

Use your horn if needed to alert other drivers or pedestrians in an emergency situation.

Road Rage –

Although it's fairly rare; also be aware of road rage and car jacking etc. Avoid getting into a confrontation with outraged drivers. Keep your doors locked in strange areas and windows rolled up to keep unwanted strangers out and again leave enough space between cars so you have an escape route if needed. Driving away to a safe area such as a police station may be your best bet. Try to get a plate number if possible and description of the vehicle.

Maneuvers You Learned But May Have Forgotten

Securing (parking) the vehicle – shift to park, apply parking brake; if uphill w/curb turn wheels to the left, if downhill or level, turn wheels to the right.

Acronyms to remember -

UCLA, which stands for uphill, curb/left always) - (DR as in doctor, which stands for downhill/right)

Backing in a straight line –

Park the car straight about six inches from the curb, line up with the curb or the car ahead of you; straighten the wheels, shift to reverse, check both mirrors and blind spots, look back to make sure there are no pedestrians, children pets or cars, lift your foot off the brake slightly and roll back at a walking speed, use the brake to control your speed, only use the gas if needed. Hold the wheel straight and make small adjustments only as needed to keep the car straight. Don't rock the wheel back and forth; this will cause you to be all over the place.

Tips –

Turn slightly to the right while moving if you need to get closer to the curb, then re straighten the wheel and continue. Remember turning right brings your back end to the right or towards the curb when backing.

Three point turn –

Remember to make three full turns – start by making one full turn to the left, check the mirror and blind spot, roll forward and stop about a foot from the curb, then make a full turn to the right, check mirror and blind spot, look back and roll back about a foot from the curb; then make a full turn left and proceed forward; remember to signal left on the first and last turns, check your left mirror and blind spot before backing, turn all the way before moving forward or back – only use as much of the road as is needed to complete your turn, watch for traffic that may try to go around you.

Five-point or Multi-point turn –

Add extra steps as needed on narrow or snow covered roads or if a parked car prohibits you from completing your three point turn safely.

Parallel Parking –

Some drivers find they are more comfortable with a three-step method and some find they like the two-step method. I suggest using the one that works for you unless you are required to use one or the other. Get use to making small adjustments by turning the wheel all the way right and inching forward to move closer to the curb or turning the wheel all the way left and inching back to get closer to the curb.

Three-step method –

Signal to pull over, line up mirror to mirror, turn the wheel one turn to the right; roll back mirror to rear bumper, then turn the wheel one turn left which straightens your wheels, roll back until your front bumper reaches the rear bumper of the parked car. Note where your right mirror lines up in relation to the parked car and use this spot as a reference point as to when to turn your wheel all the way left. Turn the wheel all the way left and roll into place. Secure the vehicle for uphill or downhill parking.

For some drivers the right side mirror should line up directly over the license plate of the parked car and for some it is slightly to the right or left. If the parked car is further from the curb then you would like to end up, bring the side mirror back a little further, a little less if the parked car is right up against the curb.

Two-step method –

This is sort of an abbreviated version of the three-step method. Signal to pull over. Line up mirror to mirror, turn one turn to the right, roll back until your front bumper lines up with the parked cars rear bumper; turn the wheel all the way left and roll back into place.

Note where your right side mirror appears to line up in relation to the parked car when you are front bumper to rear bumper and use this spot as a reference point as to when you should turn your wheel all the way left. Usually the right side mirror will appear to be over the parked car's left taillight.

Additionally, you'll need to make adjustments for example, if the car you are parking next to is a large van or pickup truck especially one with an extended cab you'll want to line up further back. Line up your passenger side mirror to his door handle or the rear door handle if it has four doors otherwise you may not have enough clearance to get around the truck as it is much longer then a midsized car. If the vehicle you are parking next to is too far from the curb, you may need to go back a little further or closer to the curb before turning your wheel all the way to the left otherwise you will be too far from the curb as well. Think of it this way; you want to do the opposite - if the parked car is too far from the curb then you need to come closer or further back; if the parked car is practically on top of the curb, you want to stay a little further away by not going back so far. If you go back too far and too close to the curb; stop and turn your wheel all the way to the right and roll forward a few inches. This will straighten the car out a few inches from the curb. If you do not have enough room to straighten out, turn the wheel all the way left and roll back a few inches this will cause the front end to move to the right or closer to the curb.

Perpendicular Parking –

Pull up perpendicular to the parking space with the space to your right side about three feet away, turn all the way left, roll forward 45-60 degrees; turn all the way right, reverse slowly, stop and straighten the wheel as car begins to straighten out, use side mirrors as needed, line up mirror to mirror or mirror to back door handle if the parked car is backed in. Use parked cars and the painted lines on the ground for references.

Things We All Should Know

1. Do a quick vehicle inspection before driving

2. Have your eyeglasses if needed for driving

3. Make sure you and all passengers have their seatbelts on

4. Know the vehicles controls

5. Take the parking brake off before proceeding

6. Signal for turns, lane changes and when pulling over to the side of the road, also on three point turns

7. Check your mirrors and blind spots when leaving the side of the road, changing lanes and backing

8. Remember to look back while backing

9. Make smooth transitions into traffic

10. Make full stops at stop signs

11. Avoid driving too fast or too slow

12. Use your horn if needed to avoid an accident or to warn pedestrians

13. No unnecessary stopping

14. Use correct lane for turns

15. Understand traffic signs

16. Know right of way rules

17. Avoid blocking crosswalks and intersections

18. Be aware of your surroundings; don't have tunnel vision

19. Yield to oncoming traffic and pedestrians

20. Avoid making fast, wide or short turns and last minute maneuvers

21. Scan intersections and roadways for traffic, pedestrians, or other hazards

22. Yield to school buses and emergency vehicles

What to do if your are involved in an automobile accident

Don't panic; have a plan!

If the unexpected happens and you are involved in a motor vehicle accident you need to:

- Call 911
- Take photos - It's important to get photos of all vehicles involved immediately after the accident to show the points of impact. Generally you'll want photos of all four corners of the car as well as close up of any damaged areas. If you can get photos of the intersection including any lights or traffic signs etc. this can help with the insurance investigation.

If a police officer is called to the scene which I recommend for even minor accidents be clear about the facts of the accident. This is your account of the accident details directly after the loss and the statements on the police report are important for your insurance company when determining which party was at fault for the accident.

Here is a list of the basic information you'll need to obtain at the accident scene. If the police were called some police reports take up to 30 days for your insurance company to obtain so it is important to gather information from the scene of the accident.

- *Date of loss*

- *Time of loss*

- *Location of the loss*

- *Conditions such as rush hour traffic, construction zone, snowstorm, heavy rain, etc.*

- *Location of loss - highway, street name, intersecting roads, shopping plaza name etc.*

- *Direction and lane of travel of your car and the other vehicles*

- *Year make, model and registration # of all cars involved*

- *Owners name and address on each car*

- *Drivers name and address and license # (if different from owners name)*

- *Insurance carrier and policy number for each car involved*

- *Name of any injured persons*

- *Name and contact number of witnesses*

Printed in Great Britain
by Amazon